TABLE OF CONTENTS

Layout and design by The Carlisle Creative LLC.
Jessica Abbott
thecarlislecreative.com

BEYOND A BITE

I'm Yaffi, registered dietitian nutritionist and food enjoyment activist, here to help you bring the joy back to your table!

This book will guide you through various activities aimed at helping increase the mindfulness factor at your dinner table (or breakfast, lunch, snack...) Aside from being a common buzzword these days, mindfulness has significant meaning and a substantial impact on how we relate to our bodies, to our food, and to our food choices.

Mindfulness is not a diet. It is not a way to manage your size or shape. It is a way to reconnect to the complete sensory experience that is food: selecting a recipe, purchasing (or growing) ingredients, preparing the food, and finally sitting down to enjoy the smells, flavors, textures, and atmosphere that make up a meal.

Mindfulness activities bring our focus back to the simple joy that is food by eliminating the "shoulds" and "what ifs" in favor of choosing to be present. Mindfulness can help you move toward a healthy relationship with food; a relationship where you can make confident decisions about your nutrition without stress or guilt, enjoying the food choices you have made, and moving on with your life after the meal has ended. This is important to both children and adults, as we often get off the path of food enjoyment. Mindfulness can be the breadcrumbs leading you back to food enjoyment.

What a wonderful gift to experience with your child.

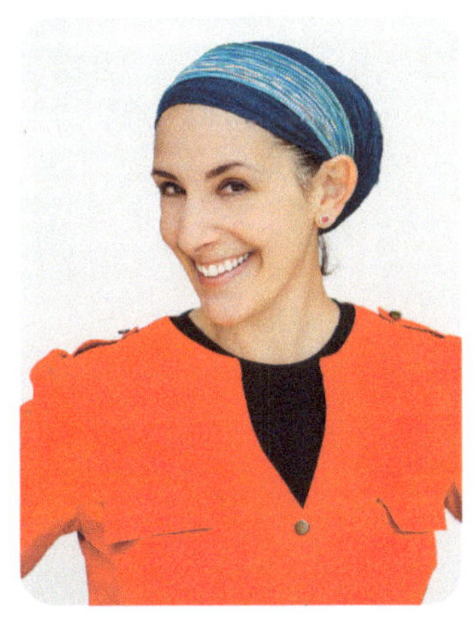

I'm Yaffi Lvova, Registered Dietitian Nutritionist and owner of Baby Bloom Nutrition® and Toddler Test Kitchen™. After studying Comparative Religions and gaining some life experience, I went back to study Nutrition and Dietetics at Arizona State University.

After a difficult journey toward and into motherhood, I became mother to twins plus one and used my experience and clinical knowledge to shift gears, providing nutrition education to new and expecting parents, with the goal of helping smooth the transition into parenthood.

In 2015, I created *Toddler Test Kitchen™* with the help of Halle Heart Children's Museum director Claudine Wessel. This unique culinary adventure puts small children in the driver's seat -- or at the cutting board as it were, helping to bolster self-esteem as they feed their curiosity by creating something delicious!

In 2016, I went live with a weekly Facebook segment and subsequent podcast, *Nap Time Nutrition©*, covering all topics parenthood and nutrition.

In 2019, I wrote *Stage-By-Stage Baby Food Cookbook: 100 Purees and Baby-Led Feeding Recipes (available in March, 2020)* and Megrette Fletcher brought me on board for the update of *Discover Mindful Eating for Kids*, continuing our mutual journey of food enjoyment activism.

This book has been reviewed by Hana Eichele, MOT, OTR/L, a Pediatric Occupational Therapist and Feeding Specialist. She is the founder and owner of Roots Pediatric Therapy, LLC, a Private Practice in Scottsdale, Arizona. Hana focuses on providing family feeding solutions to increase quality of life for the whole family! You can find Hana on Instagram at @rootspediatrictherapy

What is Mindfulness?

Mindfulness is a state of being in the present. By focusing your awareness on this very moment, while calmly acknowledging and accepting the feelings, thoughts, and experiences happening, you can create a space for breathing and for calmness.

Mindfulness helps increase trust in yourself, both in your body and in your ability to understand and make positive choices to benefit your mind, body, and spirit. Our bodies communicate basic needs through biological signals such as hunger, fullness, and satisfaction. By using mindfulness techniques at the table, we can regain trust in those signals while we help our children maintain the trust they already have in their body -- innocent trust that has been present since their birth.

How can Mindfulness Help?

Joyful time together at the dinner table together produces many benefits. According to familydinnerproject.org, benefits to family dinners include:

- Better performance in the classroom

- Increased self-esteem

- Greater sense of resilience

- Lower risk of substance abuse

- Lower risk of teen pregnancy

- Lower risk of depression

- Lower likelihood of developing eating disorders

Mindfulness can...

Help kids to stay engaged, interacting and happy, for longer amounts of time.

- Reduce parental anxiety at the table by providing a meaningful and structured activity for the whole family.

- Serve as gentle and creative nutrition exposure. Positive interactions with and around food can foster a positive relationship between mind, food choices, and body. Kids (and adults) who have this positive relationship are more likely to enjoy a wide variety of food, and therefore more likely to meet their nutrition needs for growth, development, and overall health.

• Help bring kids *(and adults too)* back in contact with their basic biological signals of hunger and fullness. This helps with both overweight and underweight concerns as the child's natural biological cues will help lead them to a healthy weight *(which doesn't look the same for all kids or adults).*

• Bolster self-esteem as children learn that they can trust their bodies and minds when making decisions. This fosters independence and confidence, skills that will carry over into interpersonal relationships, academics, and will help the child to overcome the natural obstacles that life is sure to provide.

A Few Things to Keep in Mind

The long-term goal is a child who has a healthy view of their body and is comfortable around food.

Keep this in mind.

Nutrition isn't met at a single meal or even in a single day, but over the course of a few days. The goal is to provide positive interactions with and over food.

When should you seek additional professional support? The Star Institute advises that you seek help if:

• Your child has a hard time sitting at the table for meals

• Your child eats meals separately from the rest of the family

• Your child can only eat with a distraction *(a screen, toy, or book)*

• Your child is very brand specific about which foods they will eat, or their food needs to be prepared in a very specific way

• Your child gets very upset when any new foods are presented at the meal

• Your pediatrician expresses a concern for ongoing poor weight gain *(dropping percentiles, or losing weight)*

• Your child displays frequent choking, gagging, or coughing during meals

• Your child avoids all foods of a specific texture *(crunchy foods, soft foods, purees, etc.)* or a nutrition group *(meats, fruits, vegetables, etc.)*

• Your child eats fewer than 20 foods

• Your child has a feeding tube

• Mealtimes are consistently a battle

• Your child has difficulty transitioning to solid foods *(including purees)* by 10 months, isn't accepting table foods by 12 months, is still eating only baby foods after 16 months, or hasn't transitioned to drinking something out of a cup by 16 months.

If you're working with a feeding therapist one-on-one, the advice you get from that professional will take priority over the information provided here. You can bring this to your feeding therapist as an additional resource, but advice that is specific to your family and situation is the best advice for you.

Try to have the same adventurous outlook on these activities that you are trying to help your child develop. At the same time, use your knowledge of your child to determine whether a particular activity is beneficial. Selecting and beginning an activity is not a commitment to follow through. If you try and it isn't going well, you can end the activity or take a pause and pursue another path instead.

If you are starting out with mindfulness philosophies after a history of dieting or other nutritional restriction, you may want to touch base with a non-diet registered dietitian or non-diet therapist in order to ensure the appropriate mood at the table. The goal is a child *(or adult)* who can recognize and honor their biological signals without very much thought.

If you have a child under the age of 4 years, choking hazards continue to be a concern. Avoid or modify the following foods in these activities, taken from Nationwide Children's:

• Hot dogs

• Whole nuts and seeds *(not including soft seeds such as those found in berries, zucchini, or kiwis)*

• Chunks of meat or cheese

• Whole grapes

• Hard, gooey, or sticky candy

• Popcorn

• Chunks of peanut butter or other nut or seed butter *(these ingredients can be used safely when spread thin or incorporated into baked goods)*

• Some raw produce, such as whole apples and whole carrots *(these can be modified by spiralizing or slicing into matchsticks)*

• Some dried fruit, including, but not limited to raisins, cranberries, and apricots

• Chewing gum

• Marshmallows

How Do I Use This Book?

The mindfulness activities in this book are written for ages 5 - 10. They can be adapted for younger or older children as needed -- use your knowledge of your child to create a positive experience around the table.
Remember, it's all about the smile, not the bite!

Think of these activities as gentle suggestions. Your child may opt-out the first time. That's ok. Even if it's the second or eighth time. It's very important that there is no bribing, rewarding, or punishing involved in mindfulness activities -- missing out on the fun is punishment enough!
Pick one of the following activities and just have fun with it!

Make Mealtime Enjoyable

This book is all about going Beyond a Bite by interacting with food in a positive, gentle, and creative way. Some activities can be done at the table during mealtime. Others are done as activities on their own, away from normal mealtimes and away from the dinner table.

I advocate Division of Responsibility as a positive family feeding dynamic during mealtimes. Parents are in charge of what is being served, where it is being served, and when it is being served. Children are responsible for deciding whether they will eat, and how much they will eat. For more information, visit ellynsatterinstitute.org.

• Be consistent. The location and timing of meals should be as consistent as possible. Picnics and meals out are great and should be enjoyed, but on the whole, meals should be at a predictable location *(the dinner table)* and at a predictable time.

• Proactively include a familiar food item with each meal: You can feel confident serving new *(or less-than-preferred)* food for a meal when you pair it with something your child generally accepts. Being proactive means that you decide prior to the meal what will be included rather than waiting on your child to request/demand a particular food item. The familiar food is often a carbohydrate, such as pasta or bread. It might be a PB&J sandwich. Or it might be roasted tofu. Consider the dishes your child generally requests – these are your familiar foods. The item is served as a side dish and is available to everyone at the table. If your child selects this dish and nothing else, that's perfectly fine.

Remember that the ultimate goal is a pleasant, joyful meal and that children meet their nutrition needs over a few meals or even a few days.

Say This, Not That

Instead of saying...	TRY THIS!
Clean your plate	Make your belly full
Have just one more bite	Isn't this delicious?
If you have one more bite of X, you can have dessert	If dessert is being served, it will be offered to everyone, regardless of what has or hasn't been eaten. Dessert is a family event, much like dinner, and should include everyone.
You wouldn't like it	Would you like to try a bite?
You have to try it (THE ONE BITE RULE)	Would you like to try a bite?
I'm so glad you ate that!	I'm so proud of your bravery! It's fun to try new foods!
(Toward another person) "Daniel is so picky. He wouldn't eat that."	"Daniel is learning to like new foods."
Mommy doesn't like mushrooms	Avoid calling attention to what is or isn't on your own plate or on someone else's plate. If the child asks about it, you can say, "Mushrooms aren't my taste, but Daddy loves them! I wonder what you think. Do you want to try?"
What do you want to eat?	You, the parent or caretaker, are responsible for making decisions concerning what is being served. At snack time, you may give a choice between two acceptable options: "Would you rather have crackers or pretzels?" or "Would you rather have an apple or an orange?" At breakfast, lunch, and dinner, the parent or caretaker decides what will be offered, places it on the table, and the child may choose from what has been made available to them.

More Table Tips

LOOK UP, NOT DOWN!

Mealtime is a wonderful opportunity to enjoy your child's company. When you focus on their plate -- on how many bites they have eaten or what they decided not to select -- you miss an opportunity for meaningful engagement. Look at your child's face, at their smile. Listen to what is important for them to share and participate in a conversation on their level. The confidence boost they get from this attention will make this mealtime more pleasant, but will also carry over to future mealtimes -- they will approach the table with confidence in the knowledge that you want to spend quality time with them.

SPEAK TO YOUR CHILD AS YOU WOULD SPEAK TO A GUEST AT YOUR TABLE.

Before you ask your child to "Take just one more bite" or "Eat three bites of broccoli and you can have ice cream," consider whether or you would say this to a guest at your table. Would you assume that you know exactly how full your guest is? When visiting a friend's table, would you consider it appropriate for your friend to offer dessert or not based on how many bites you had consumed? Consider your child a guest at your table and treat them as such. While they may still need help cutting their food or wiping up a spill, it's important to recognize that your child is an independent person with their own feelings -- both physical and emotional -- trying to spend quality time with you while independently meeting their own needs -- again, both physical and emotional. You can encourage that independence by limiting comments to the respectful, the funny, and the supportive types of comments you would make to a guest at your table.

DON'T YUCK MY YUM!

Most people have something that they dislike, often something that many other people love to eat. Children are finding their own way through their flavor preferences. During this journey, they may do something we find to be unpalatable. They may dip their banana in ketchup, for example. When we allow children to find their own way, without imposing our own flavor preferences on them, we are also teaching them that different people like different flavors, and that's ok. This can lead to conversations about how people around the world eat differently, using different utensils and different flavor combinations.

WHEN TRYING SOMETHING NEW...

The child may feel more adventurous if they sit on the parent's lap while trying something new. Trying a bite of something off the parent's fork is much less intimidating than having it on their own plate. The offer must be made in a neutral way: "Would you like to try a bite from my fork?" rather than, "Just try a bite."

SELECTIVE ("PICKY") EATING IS A PHASE.

My great-grandmother used to say, "Don't create a problem where there isn't one." Selective ("picky") eating is a normal, natural phase. Continue to offer a variety of foods through this time in order to maximize exposure. The more often a child comes in contact with a particular food, the more familiar it becomes and the more likely they are to be comfortable with it.

Toddlers very often choose to be vegetarian. If the family is not vegetarian, the parents may choose to offer meats that are wetter in nature -- stews, meatballs in sauce, and many slow cooker or pressure cooker recipes tend to go over well with these children.

Skipping dinner is also a common, and natural occurrence in children. They can certainly meet their nutrition needs while missing one meal. If there is a 2-3 hour gap between dinner and bedtime, it is appropriate to offer a snack before bedtime, regardless of whether they ate dinner or not.

It is also common for young children to limit their list of acceptable foods, particularly between the ages of 12 and 24 months. Continue to offer a variety. If their "acceptable foods" list becomes shorter and shorter, you may seek one on one help from a non-diet pediatric dietitian.

ALLOW THE CHILD TO SERVE HIM OR HERSELF, FAMILY-STYLE

From a very young age, children are able to indicate whether or not they would like to enjoy a particular food during mealtime. Younger children can point, smile, and giggle, while older children can fully serve themselves. Maximize their independence by allowing them to serve themselves as early as possible.

SERVING SIZES

The appropriate serving size for your child is the size of their fist. Encourage children to take roughly that amount of each desired food, reminding them that they will be able to take as much as they need to fill their bellies. Small portions reduce overwhelm at the table while also limiting food waste. The child should be allowed to have seconds, thirds, or even fifths as needed/desired.

LISTEN TO YOUR CHILD

Your child's biological signals of hunger and fullness are as valid as yours are. They know how to recognize and communicate their needs from the time they are born. Listen to your child. Offer meals and snacks no more than 2-3 hours apart, and listen to them when they say they are hungry or full. You never know when a big milestone, a cold, or a growth spurt is around the corner.

OFFER SWEETS

Many parents try to avoid sweets in an effort to promote preference for more savory foods. This can backfire as sugary foods get that delicious "forbidden fruit" label. By exposing children to sweets, by going on family trips for ice cream or enjoying French toast with maple syrup together, the idea of sugary foods is neutralized and becomes less alluring.

EATING OUT

Going out to eat with small children can be a real challenge. Minimize the obstacles by selecting a family-friendly restaurant, calling ahead to order, and serving food in the same way that you do at home. Instead of choosing one entree per person, choose a couple of appetizers and a couple of main dishes (from the adult menu) and share, family-style.

BE PREDICTABLE
Follow a predictable schedule and serve food in a predictable location. Children find comfort in routine.

THINK BEYOND THE TABLE
Food exposure doesn't only happen at mealtime but occurs the grocery store, while looking at the recipe book, cooking together, making food art, or even coloring in pictures of food (check out Let's Play with Our Food: My Fruit and Veggie Coloring Book by Dani Lebovitz). Consider starting an herb garden or visiting a local farm that offers You-Pick.

EMPLOY POSITIVE PARENTING TECHNIQUES
Positive Parenting is a gentle technique that encourages bonding and independence by establishing realistic and appropriate boundaries in a positive way. For more information, I encourage you to visit @unconditional_parenting on Instagram.

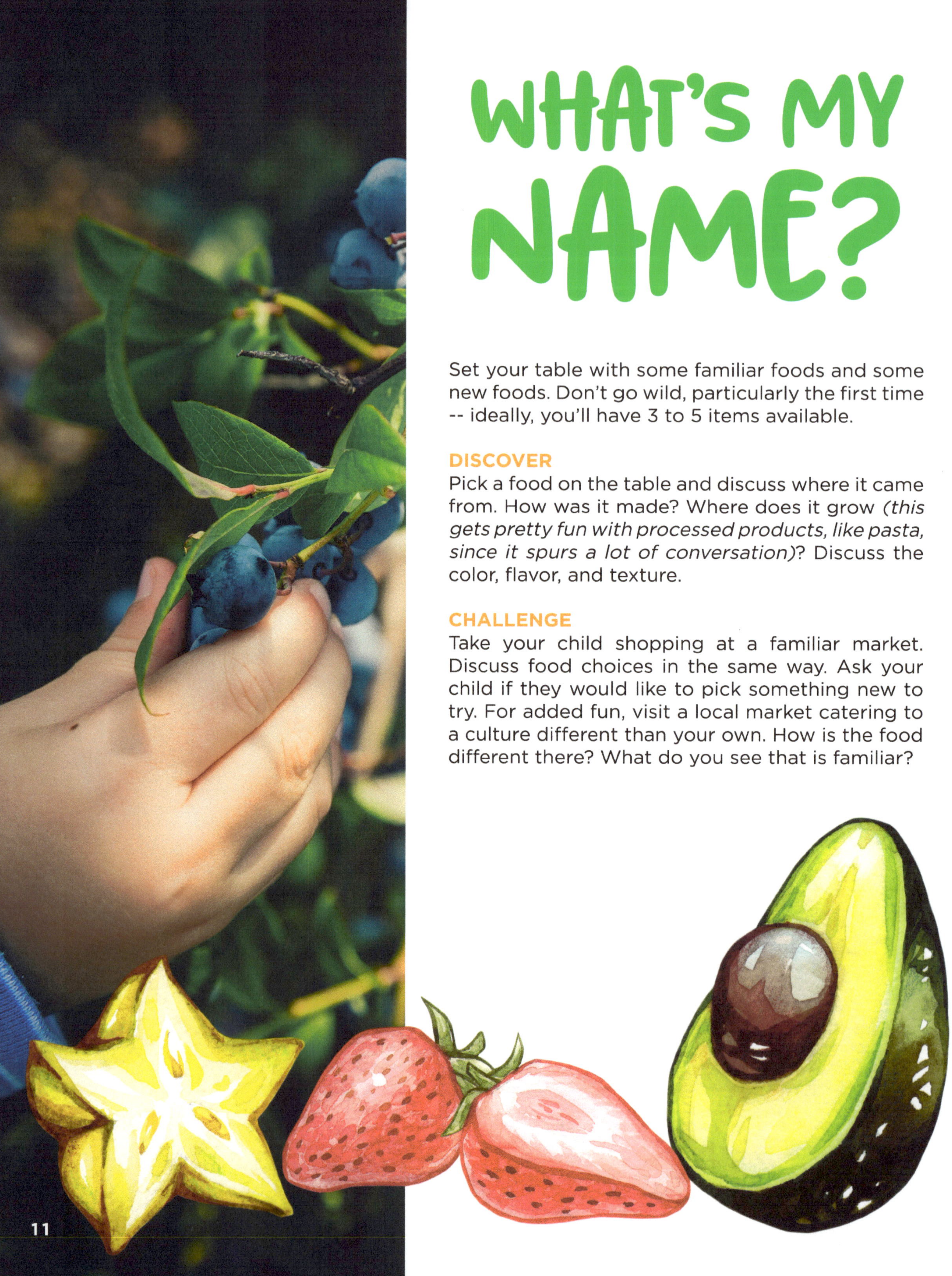

WHAT'S MY NAME?

Set your table with some familiar foods and some new foods. Don't go wild, particularly the first time -- ideally, you'll have 3 to 5 items available.

DISCOVER
Pick a food on the table and discuss where it came from. How was it made? Where does it grow (this gets pretty fun with processed products, like pasta, since it spurs a lot of conversation)? Discuss the color, flavor, and texture.

CHALLENGE
Take your child shopping at a familiar market. Discuss food choices in the same way. Ask your child if they would like to pick something new to try. For added fun, visit a local market catering to a culture different than your own. How is the food different there? What do you see that is familiar?

1, 2, 3, CRUNCH!

Set out a bowl of crunchy veggies in the middle of the table *(such as carrots, peppers, celery sticks, cucumber spears or rounds, sugar snap peas, jicama, etc.)* Be sure to have at least three options, ideally different in color from each other. You'll want to keep in mind any choking hazards if you have a child under the age of four years. If this is a new activity for your little one, consider having a delicious dip handy as well. Some great options are guacamole, hummus, tzatziki, roasted vegetable dip, or this delicious vegan queso.

DISCOVER
Choose an item from your Crunch Bowl. What color is this? What else is the same color? Where does this grow? What else grows the same way? Do you think it will be loud? Soft? How will it taste? Sweet? Bitter? Do you want to dip it?

PLAY
Everyone grabs a crunchy veggie. Hold up your crunch of choice, count to three together and crunch at the same time.

CHALLENGE
Kick it up a notch!

- Discuss who made the loudest crunch.

- Encourage your child to cover their ears as they crunch down -- ask if this made their crunch super quiet or super loud!

- Ask your child to crunch on the right side. On the left side. With their front teeth. With their back teeth. Does it sound different? Does it taste different?

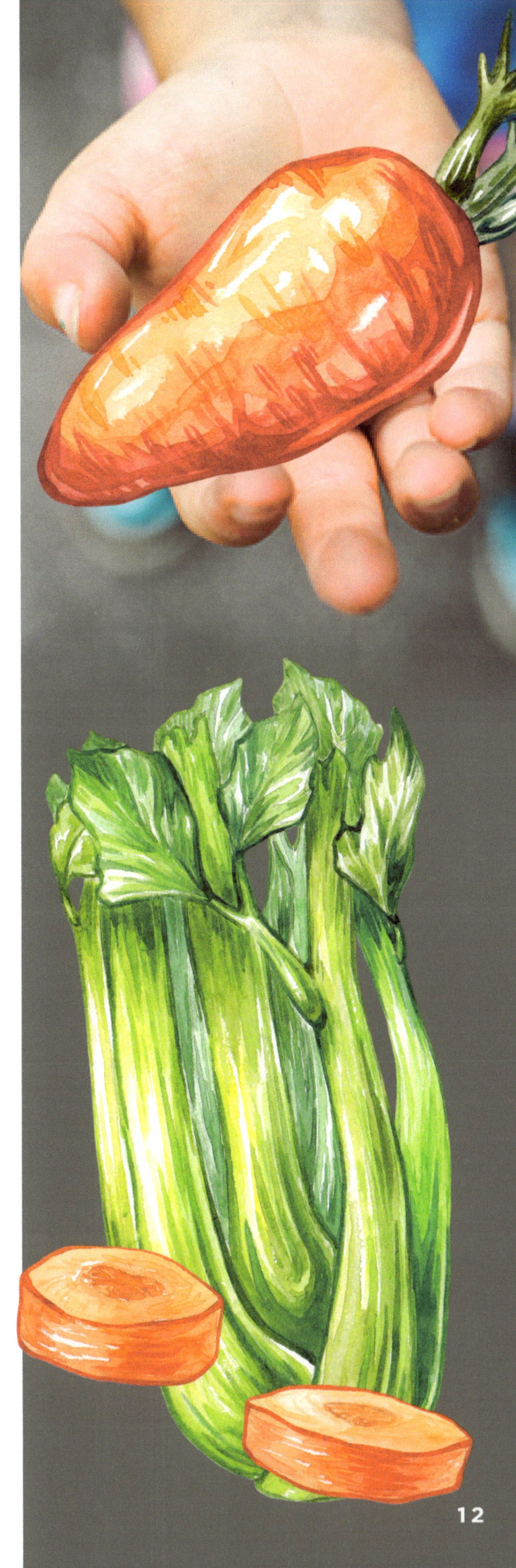

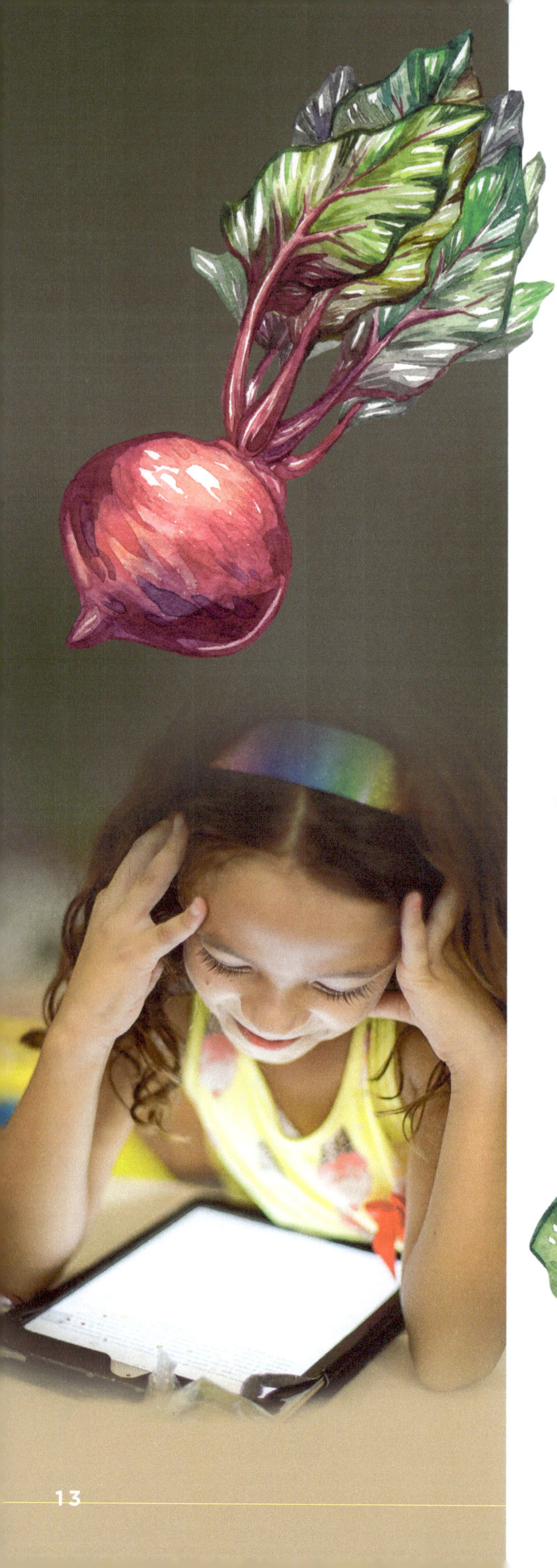

DO DRAGONS EAT BROCCOLI?

DISCOVER

Pick an item of food that you're planning to serve with dinner. Search YouTube for "animal eating broccoli" *(or whichever food you have selected)*. Cuddle up on the couch with your mini-me, watch, and discuss. Was it cute? Sloppy or neat? Did the animal enjoy the food? Is this a food the animal can easily and regularly access?

PLAY

Move your party to the table. Ask your child, "How would a *[goldfish/hamster/dragon]* eat this? Do you want to show me?" If the child isn't interested, show off your own imitation skills. The goofier, the better.

CHALLENGE

Discuss tonight's dinner plan with your child and have them select a food for this activity. Which food would be the most fun? The messiest? The tiniest? The biggest?

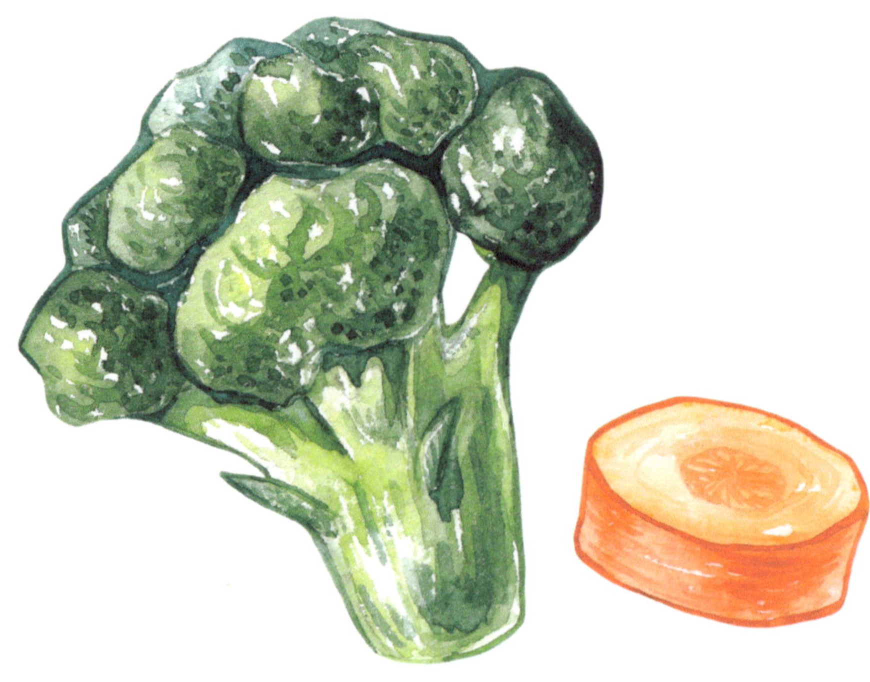

HOW FULL is YOUR BELLY?

Print out a basic image of the digestive tract. Discuss the different parts of the digestive tract with your child. This doesn't have to be complex. Ask them to point out where the esophagus is on their own body. Where is your stomach? Where are your intestines? You can discuss what each part does, getting more specific as the child grows. A conversation with a 3-year-old might look like this:

• Food travels down the esophagus into the stomach.

• The stomach churns the food, like a blender, before sending it into the intestines.

• Food that isn't needed comes out as poop! *(Kids particularly love that part.)*

The same conversation with a 10-year-old would get a bit deeper.

• After chewing, saliva helps the food move down the esophagus in a movement that looks like an inchworm moving *(you can watch a video on this too)*. Each bite, called a bolus, mixes with saliva and moves down the esophagus toward the stomach.

• As the food moves into the stomach, there is a cap that closes on the top of the stomach and one on the bottom so that food stays in the stomach. The walls of the stomach look like a washboard to help mash up the food while stomach acid cleans off the food so it's safe to eat.

• Food moves into the small intestine where micronutrients such as vitamins and minerals are absorbed into the body.

• Food then moves from the small intestine into the large intestine where water is absorbed.

• Unused food is then eliminated as poop. *(This continues to be amusing.)*

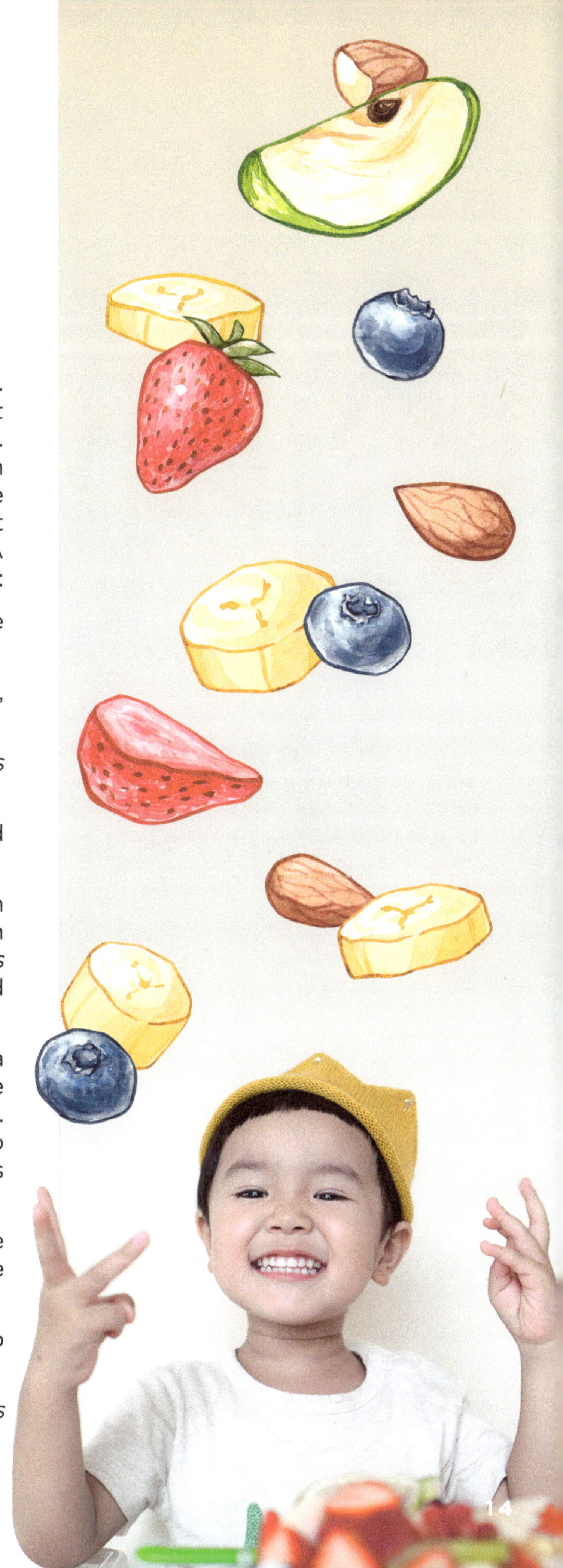

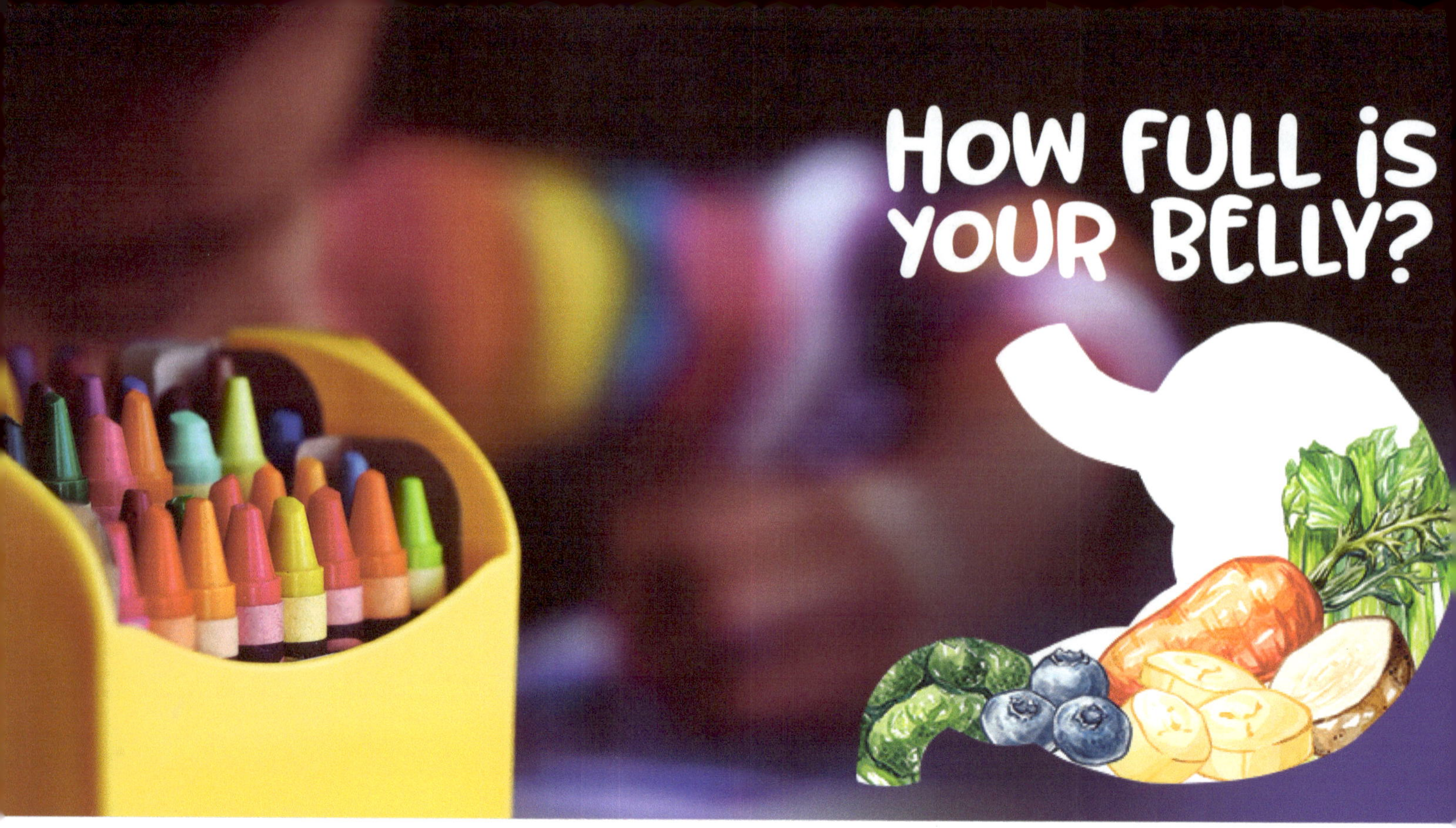

HOW FULL is YOUR BELLY?

PLAY

During mealtime, give your child a piece of paper with the general shape of the stomach on it as well as a crayon. Take a tummy-check break during your meal, like a seventh inning stretch, and ask them to color in how full their belly is in that moment. After coloring, return to the meal and continue.

IMPORTANT NOTES

This is a zero-judgment game. All of these activities are zero-judgment games. Allow your child to show you their picture and explain how full their belly is. Refrain from commenting yourself on how much they have already eaten or how much you believe they should eat. This activity is merely to bring the child back into contact with the basic biological signals of hunger and fullness. It is of utmost importance that the child understands that there will be enough food to make a full belly.

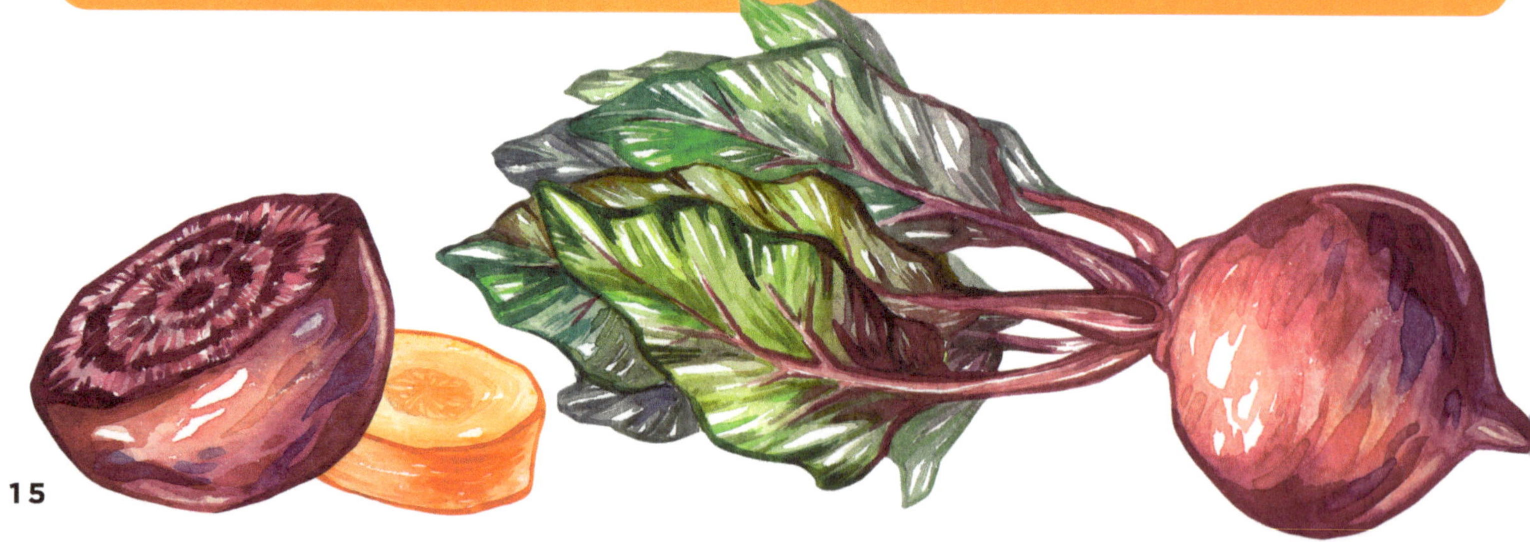

SUPERHERO DINNER

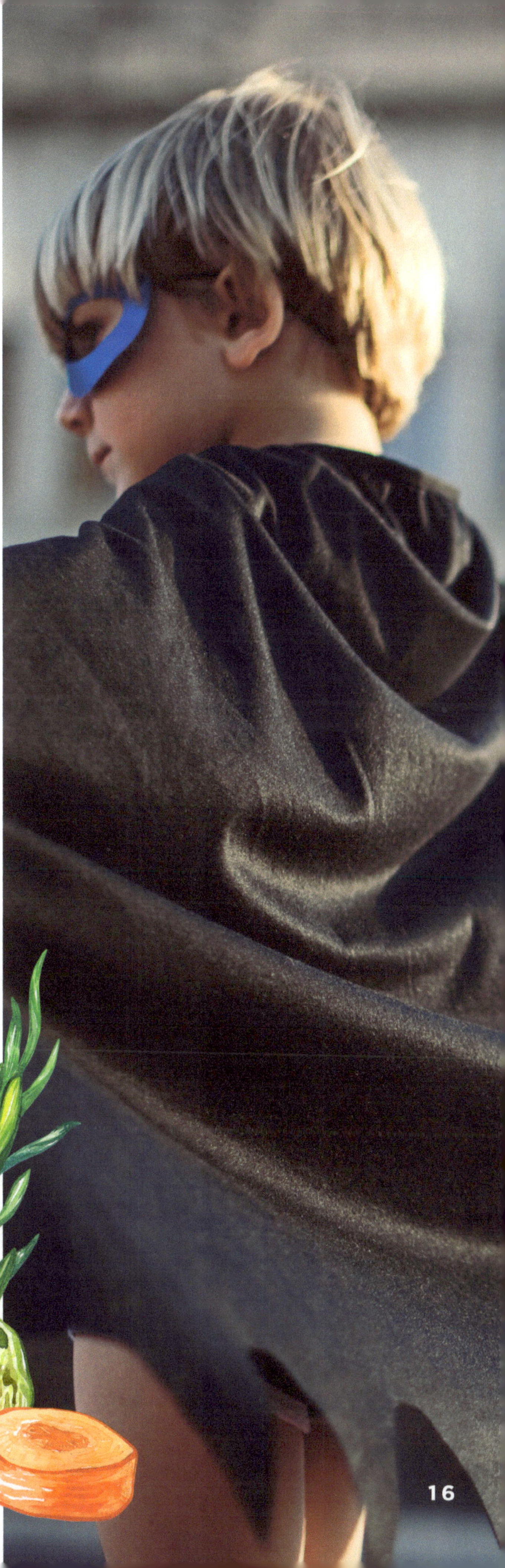

DISCOVER

Ask your child who their favorite superhero or cartoon character is. Prompt your child to explain to you why this character is their favorite and what extraordinary abilities they may have. Request an impression of the character if your child is very interested in this discussion.

PLAY

Serve dinner for the whole family on Wonder Woman-themed plates *(or whomever your child has described)* and ask your child if the food tastes extra-super. How would that superhero eat their dinner? Fast? Slow? What do you think their favorite food is?

CHALLENGE

If you have more than one child, ask one to pick their sibling's favorite theme as a surprise.

IMPORTANT NOTES

It's very easy to go full-on birthday mode with this one. Try to keep it simple. Sensory overwhelm can negatively impact appetite. Themed plates, cups, and/or napkins is sufficient. Balloons can be distracting.

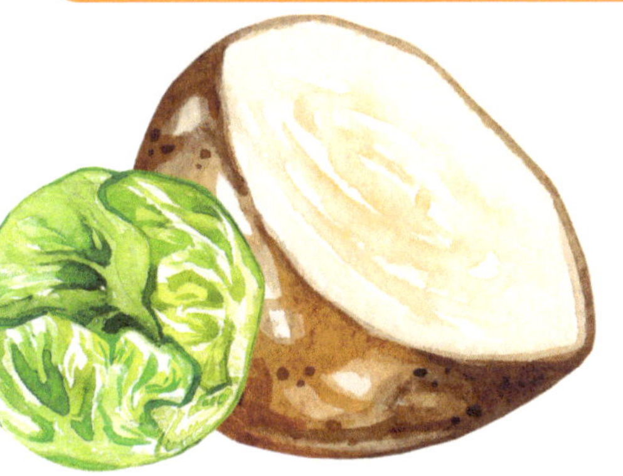

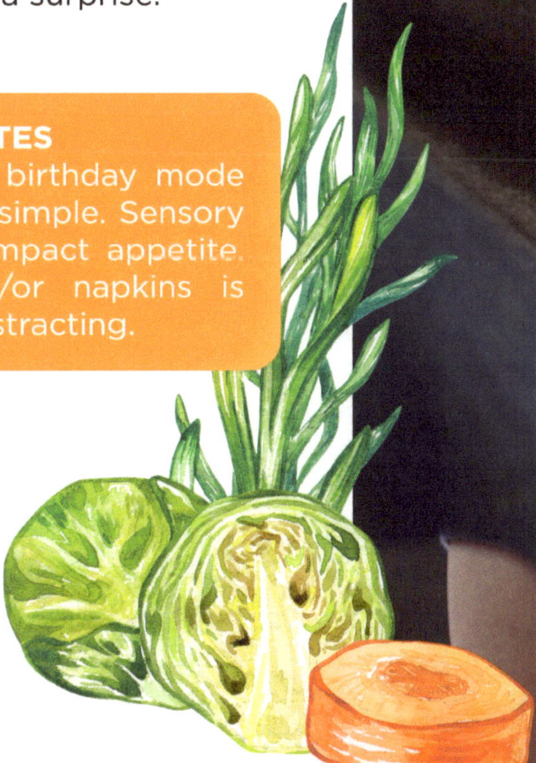

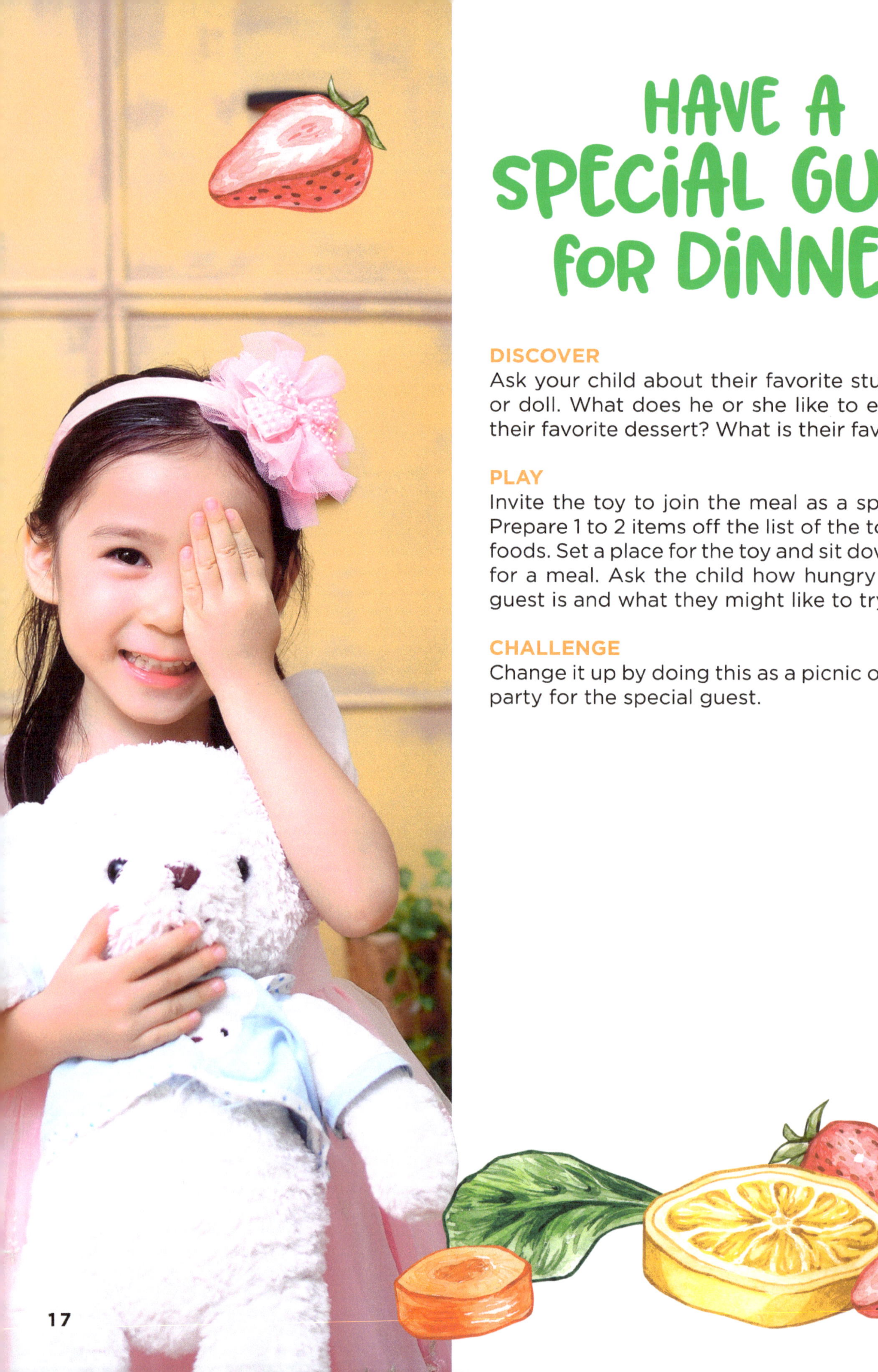

HAVE A SPECIAL GUEST FOR DINNER

DISCOVER

Ask your child about their favorite stuffed animal or doll. What does he or she like to eat? What is their favorite dessert? What is their favorite color?

PLAY

Invite the toy to join the meal as a special guest. Prepare 1 to 2 items off the list of the toy's favorite foods. Set a place for the toy and sit down together for a meal. Ask the child how hungry the special guest is and what they might like to try today.

CHALLENGE

Change it up by doing this as a picnic or a birthday party for the special guest.

SIBLING TRANSLATION

DISCOVER

One of the most fun parts of parenting has been seeing my kids become big brothers. When their little brother is having a tantrum, I can ask his big brothers for translation. This can help at mealtimes as well. But please note: don't use this one very often. Once in a while is novel. More frequent use could cause strain between siblings.

PLAY

Ask one child, "How hungry is your brother/sister?" This is just to spur conversation around appetite. "Does he/she have a big appetite?", "Does he/she have a little appetite?"

CHALLENGE

Take this to the next level by doing it game-show style. Ask the following questions, or equally neutral questions you may come up with, and then ask the smaller child if their bigger sibling was correct.

- "What is your sibling's favorite food?"

- "What is your sibling's favorite meal of the day?"

- "What is your sibling's favorite crunchy/creamy/ sweet food?"

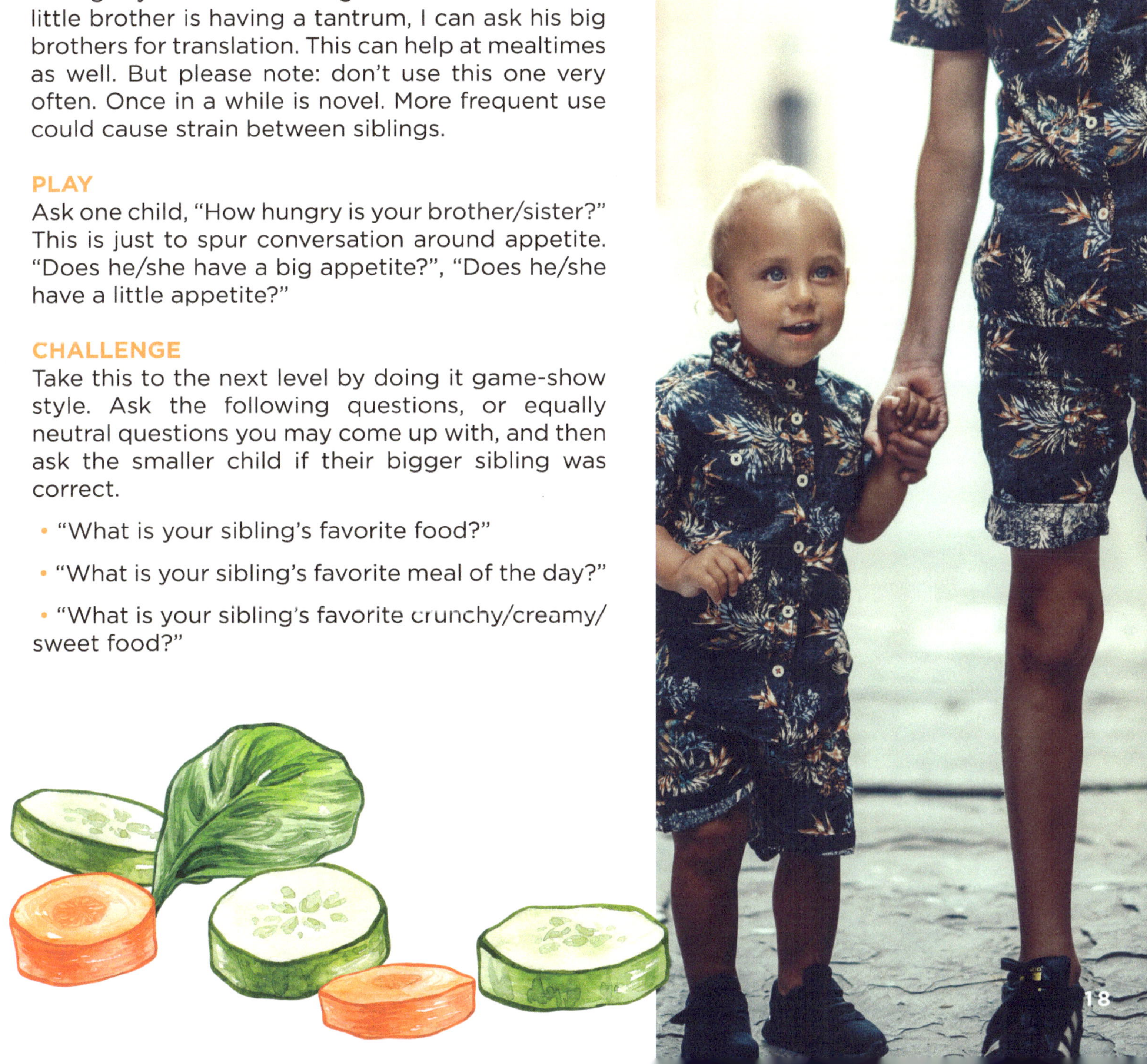

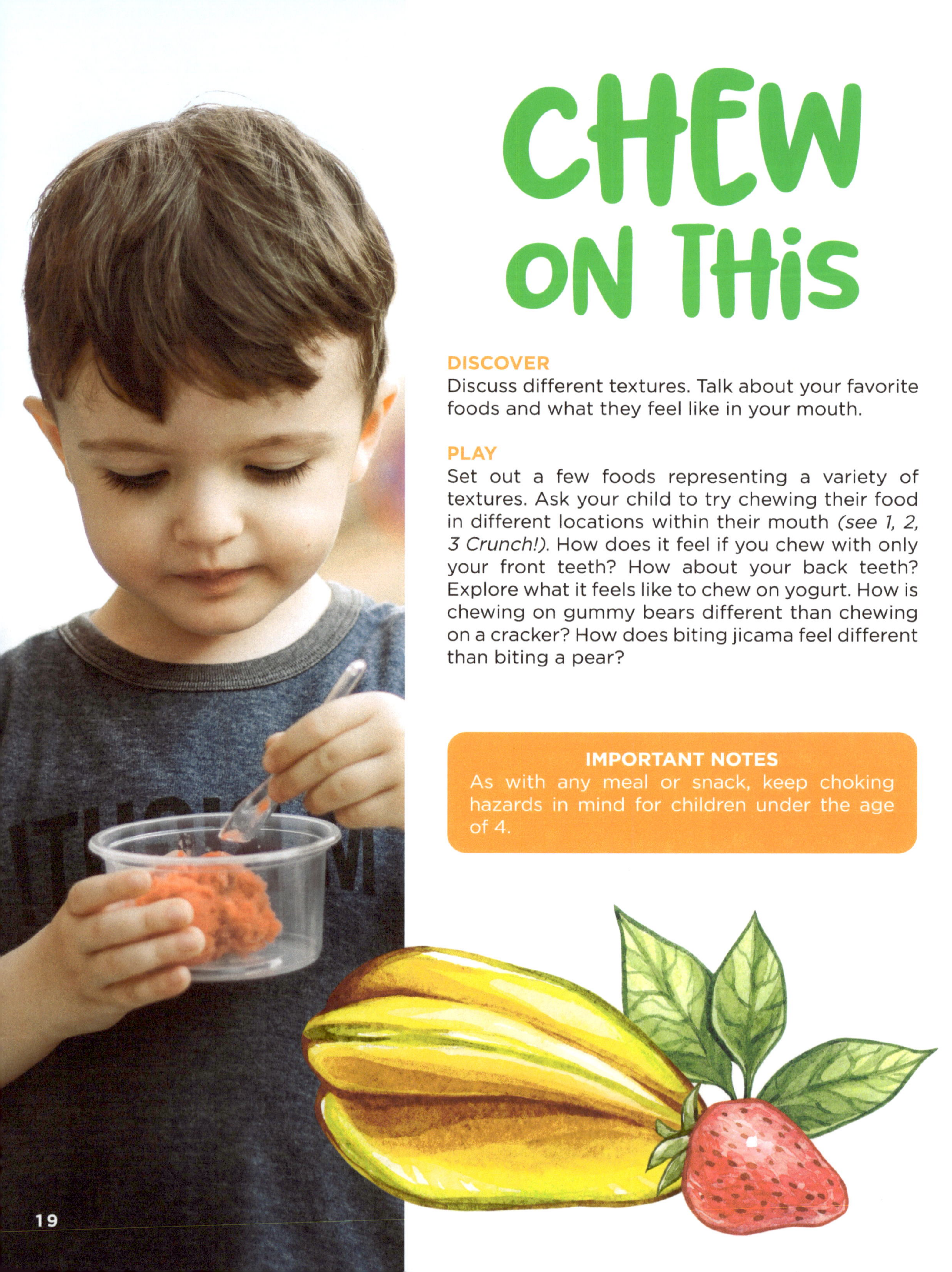

CHEW ON THIS

DISCOVER

Discuss different textures. Talk about your favorite foods and what they feel like in your mouth.

PLAY

Set out a few foods representing a variety of textures. Ask your child to try chewing their food in different locations within their mouth *(see 1, 2, 3 Crunch!)*. How does it feel if you chew with only your front teeth? How about your back teeth? Explore what it feels like to chew on yogurt. How is chewing on gummy bears different than chewing on a cracker? How does biting jicama feel different than biting a pear?

IMPORTANT NOTES

As with any meal or snack, keep choking hazards in mind for children under the age of 4.

A FORK BY ANY OTHER NAME

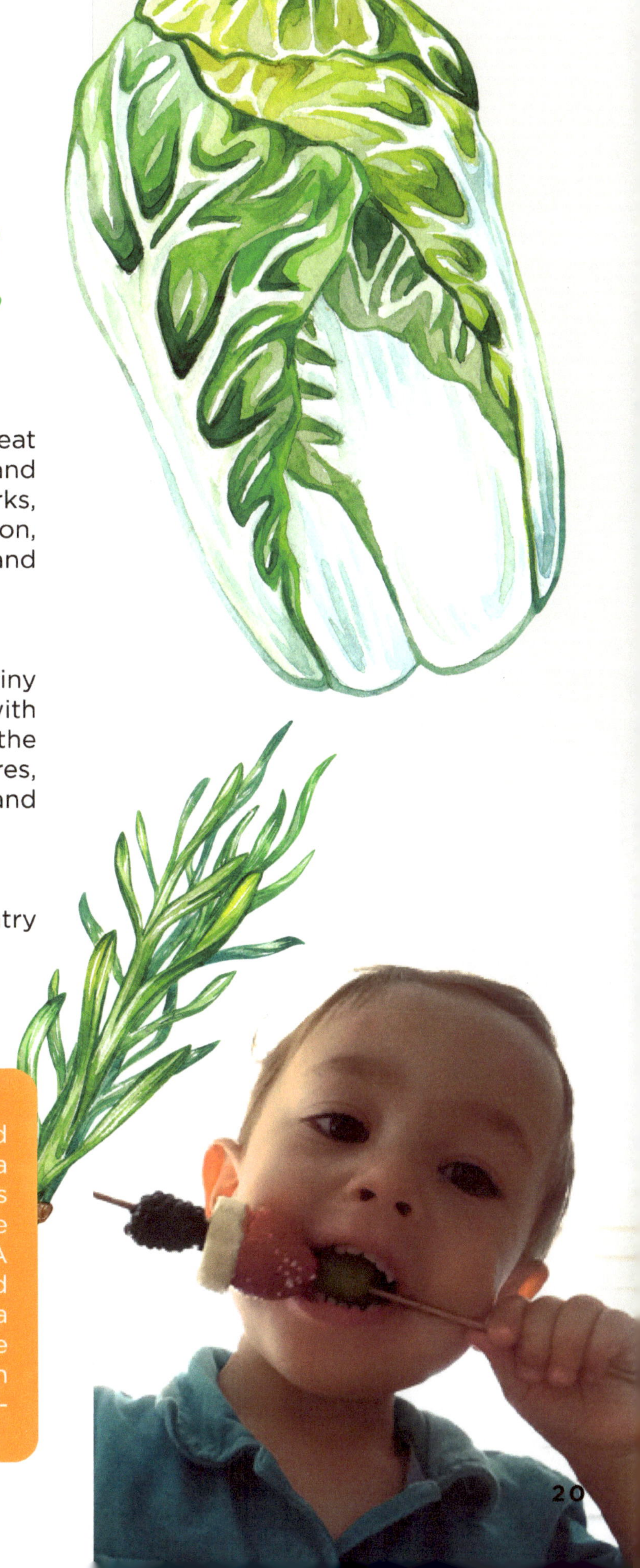

DISCOVER

Discuss how people around the world eat differently. Use a world map for inspiration, and go to YouTube for videos on eating with forks, chopsticks, sporks, and more. For inspiration, google "eating utensils around the world" and "unusual eating utensils

PLAY

Use alternative utensils, such as mini tongs, tiny forks, child-safe toothpicks, or chopsticks (with chopstick helpers). You can often find these at the dollar store, international markets, party stores, or you can visit my Pinterest board Books and Gadgets at Pinterest.com/yaffi.

CHALLENGE

Add to the fun by playing music from the country where the selected utensil is popular.

IMPORTANT NOTES

Always be sure to serve a familiar food alongside anything new, particularly with a hesitant or selective (picky) eater. This helps boost the confidence they will need to be adventurous with their food selections. A hesitant eater may prefer to try a new food while sitting on a parent's lap or by eating a bite from the parent's plate since it feels like less commitment on the child's part. You can also offer a no-thank-you plate for less-than-successful bites.

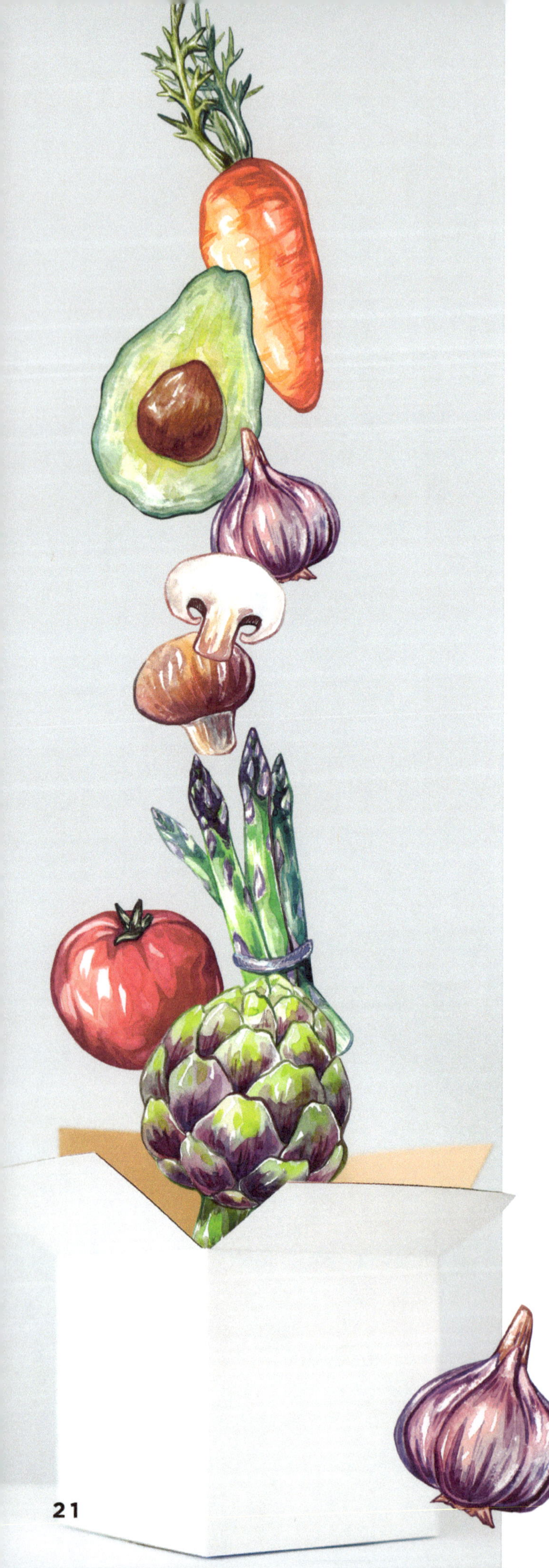

WHAT'S IN THE BOX?

DISCOVER

Ask your child what their favorite fruit is. Vegetable? Type of pasta (in color, size, and shape)? Dip? Do they prefer hot or cold? Take these suggestions, pair them with some unfamiliar foods, and use them for this fun activity.

Please note:
This may not be appropriate for children with more intense sensory processing concerns.

PLAY

Get an empty shoebox *(or a few if they are available)*. Cut a fist-size circle through the top of the lid. Place the food item in the box. Ask your child for permission to use a blindfold. Then, either blindfold your child, or if that makes them nervous, ask them to look away from the box *(if that also makes them nervous, see Important Notes below)*. Ask them to feel the food inside the box - how does it feel? Do you know what it is? Have them place a surprise food in the box for you to identify!

IMPORTANT NOTES

If you begin this activity and your child appears nervous or otherwise distressed, you can either pursue a different activity, or you can do away with the box and simply discuss how the no-longer-mystery food feels in their hand. It's very important to remain neutral if the activity isn't working out for your child. Sometimes we all just need a change in direction.

Resources

Stacking your social media feed with reliable information can be a big help when navigating parenthood. Here are some accounts I think you should follow for great info!

@adolescent.nutritionist

@amyreednutrition

@bodypositive_mom

@dianakrice

@drjencohen

@equal.parenting.nutrition

@experience.delicious

@family.snack.nutritionist

@feedingbliss

@feedinglittles

@fromatozucchini

@healthymomma_healthykids

@lnznutrition

@mamaandsweetpea

@momntotnutrition

@natalia.stasenko

@nutritionhungry

@nutritioninbloom

@rootspediatrictherapy

@thedoctorandthedietitian

@thefamilykitchencoach

@tinybitesnutrition

@toddler.testkitchen
(that's me!)

Nutrition for Raising Children

Naptimenutrition.com: You can find me here, weekly, giving free and up to date information on parenting, children, and nutrition. Use the search tab to explore topics I've covered since 2016: gluten, fat, pumping, how to read growth charts, and so much more! You can also find limited *(but growing!)* Nap Time Nutrition segments as a podcast on Apple, Spotify, and Stitcher.

Babybloomnutrition.com: Also me! Join my Save My Sanity course -- nutritional confidence for the whole family!

Baby-led Weaning Resources

FeedingLittles.com: Feeding Littles has wonderful online courses in both Baby-led Weaning and Toddler Feeding. You can use the code BABYBLOOM to get 10% off either of those courses.

Stage-By-Stage Baby Food Cookbook: 100 Purees and Baby-Led Feeding Recipes *(available in March, 2020 on amazon.com)*

Baby-led Weaning Cookbook: This is a great resource for both information on Baby-led Weaning and delicious recipes for the whole family.

Child Nutrition Resources

Ellynsatterinstitute.org: Ellyn Satter, MS, RD, MSSW developed the Division of Responsibility positive child feeding model. Her site is a valuable resource for further information on guiding your child toward a healthy relationship with food and body.

FeedingBytes.com: Natalia Stasenko, RD and feeding expert provides up to date and convenient resources on her site as well on her social media outlets.

Thefeedingdoctor.com: Katja Rowell, MD provides books, blogs, and other free resources on child nutrition, extreme picky eating, food preoccupation, and much more.

Healthychildren.org: The American Academy of Pediatrics has a parenting website. You can visit this site to get reliable health information concerning parenting and children.

Babywearing Resources

Tandemtrouble.com: LaKeta Kemp, babywearing coach and twin mom (like me!) demonstrates how to wear twins safely and comfortably.

Breastfeeding Resources

Ilca.org: International Lactation Consultants Association has a search function to help connect you with an international board certified lactation consultant (IBCLC). Having an advocate during this amazing time can provide important relief.

Crystalkarges.com and **mamaandsweetpeanutrition.com**: Find reliable and compassionate advice on breastfeeding and breastfeeding nutrition from these two registered dietitians.

Sleep Resources

Getquietnights.com: Tracy Spackman provides gentle sleep coaching information. Check out her blog for daily schedules, including alternative options.

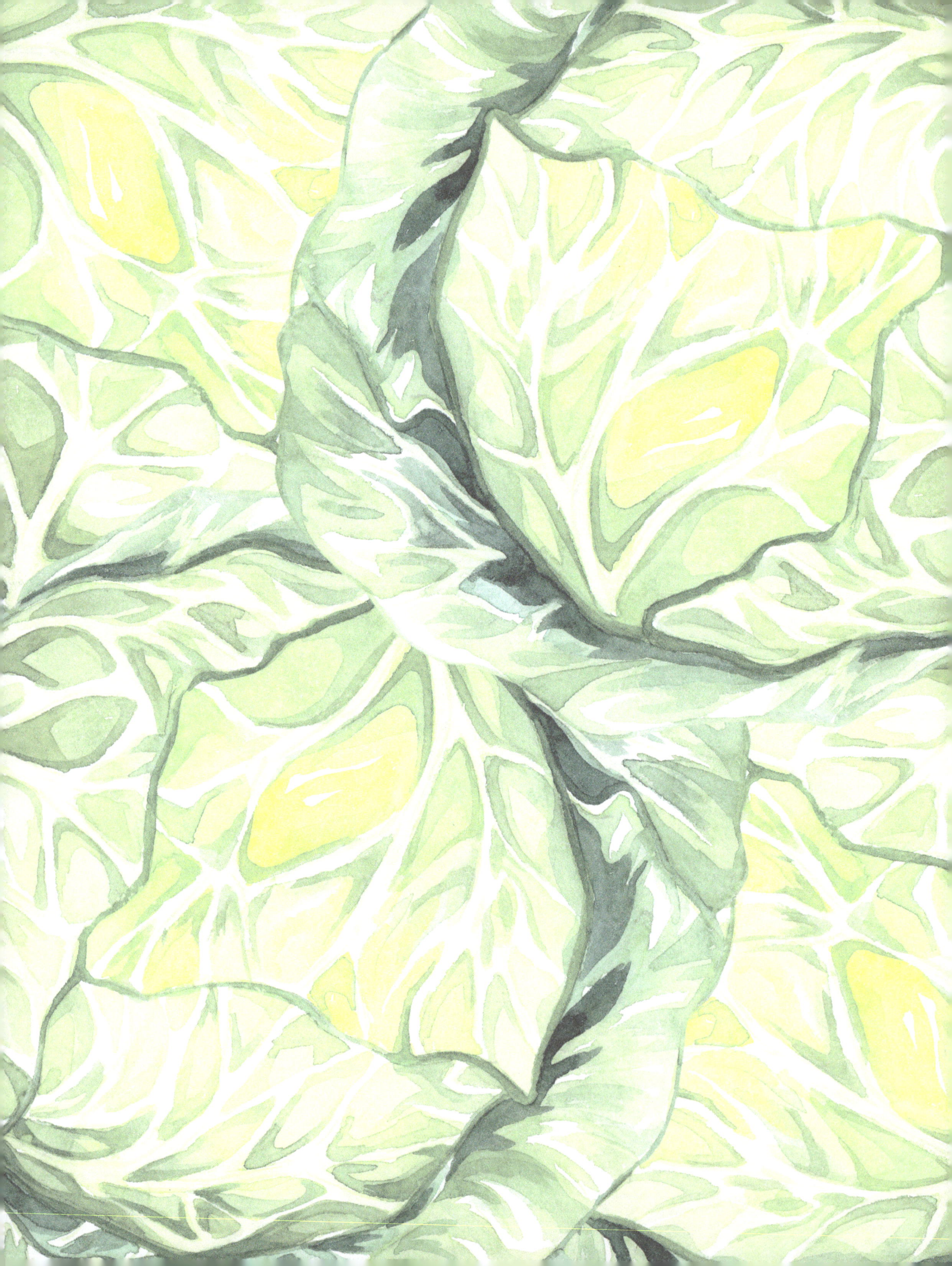